Y0-DYM-450

Hospital

Administration

Terminology

American Hospital Association
840 North Lake Shore Drive
Chicago, Illinois 60611

Library of Congress Cataloging in Publication Data
Main entry under title:

Hospital administration terminology

"AHA catalog no. 001110."
    1. Hospitals--Dictionaries. 2. Hospitals--Administra-
tion--Dictionaries. 3. Medical care--Dictionaries.
I. American Hospital Association. [DNLM: 1. Hospital
administration--Terminology. WX 13 H828]
RA962.2.H67   362.1 '1 '068   82-6782
ISBN 0-87258-367-8   AACR2

AHA catalog no. 001110

Preface

This alphabetical glossary contains terms that have application to the administration of hospitals and related health care institutions and to health care delivery in general. Although other definitions may be used in the hospital administration field and although regional or other variations may be in use, the terms selected are those considered most commonly used by and most useful to hospital administrators.

Terms that have application beyond the health care field—for example, chaplain—are defined here in the hospital context. The occupational terms listed are not intended to be job descriptions, so details of job duties and responsibilities are deliberately omitted.

The book does not include clinical and technical terms used primarily by specialized departments or terms related to the practice of medicine per se. For example, terms related to antibiotics and equipment are not included.

Throughout the book, the word *hospital* is used in a generic sense to refer to any health care institution. This is an editorial convenience to save space and avoid repetition. When the word *hospital* is used, the reader should substitute, as appropriate, nursing home, satellite clinic, ambulatory care facility, or other health care institution.

Considerable effort was made to be as concise as possible without sacrificing accuracy and to make the definitions of similar and related terms as consistent as possible. The definition is given with the term that is most generally accepted; alternative terms are appropriately cross-referenced.

Because the terms are subject to change as hospital care itself changes, the book is not intended to be definitive or all-inclusive. Further, this book is not intended as a legal reference. Many of the terms listed have specific and limited meaning in various legal contexts. The definitions used in this book relate to common usage and not to specific legal meanings.

Readers with suggestions for revisions or additions are encouraged to send them to the American Hospital Association, Division of Books and Newsletters, 840 N. Lake Shore Dr., Chicago, IL 60611.

Acknowledgments

A publication of this scope could not have been undertaken without the contributions of many specialists at the American Hospital Association as well as other hospital-related organizations.

The contributions of staff of the following organizations in reviewing definitions related to their fields of interest are gratefully acknowledged:

American Association of Blood Banks, Stephanie Summers
American Association of Nurse Anesthetists, Josephine Heimler
American College of Hospital Administrators, Carrol Micky
American College of Obstetricians and Gynecologists,
  Warren E. Pearse, M.D.
American Dental Association, Louis Joseph
American Medical Technologists, Chester Dziekonski
American Society of Hospital Pharmacists, James Caro
Centers for Disease Control, U.S. Department of Health and Human
  Services, Richard E. Dixon, M.D.
College of American Pathologists, Pam Cramer
Hospital Financial Management Association, James T. Whitman and
  James Bollinger

The assistance of the following present and former AHA staff members is also gratefully acknowledged: Catherine Begole, Ruth Behrens, Edward Bertz, Linda Burns, Mary Converse, Richard diMonda, Betty Dudley, Alice Dunlap, Mindy Ferber, Conn Flatley, Susan Fort, Alex Gekas, Joan Gilmour, Lawrence Goldberg, James Groves, Michael Guerin, John Hatfield, Jay Hedgepeth, Betty Kojima, Peter Kralovec, Carol Lively, Karen Longo, Julie Manez, Brandon Melton, Bonnie Miller, Shirley Ann Munroe, Nancie Noie, Salie Rossen, Arline Sax, David Schaeffer, Victoria Smaller, and Richard Umbdenstock.

Special appreciation is expressed to Helen D. Hunt, for providing leadership and direction during the developmental stages of the project; to Sharyn Sweeney Bills, for researching and writing the majority of the definitions; to Madison B. Brown, M.D., for reviewing the manuscript and making valuable suggestions for revision; to Rex N. Olsen, for his guidance and support throughout the project. Editorial services were provided by Louise Mirkin and Carl V. Boyer, under the direction of Dorothy Saxner, director, Division of Books and Newsletters.

Aa

absence, day on leave of 24-hour interval of an authorized absence of an inpatient

accreditation formal process of evaluation and recognition that an institution or educational or training program meets the standards of an accrediting organization

accredited formally recognized by an accrediting organization as meeting its standards

accredited hospital See *hospital, accredited*

activities therapist See *therapeutic recreation specialist*

acute disease disease characterized by a single episode of fairly short duration, usually less than 30 days, and from which the patient can be expected to return to his or her normal or previous state and level of activity

acute hospital See *hospital, short-term*

administrative adjustment bookkeeping adjustment to reflect services provided but not billed to patients because costs of billing and collection would exceed charges, or to reflect partial adjustment of charges in special circumstances

administrative engineer See *engineer, administrative*

administrator See *chief executive officer*

admission formal acceptance by a hospital of a patient who is to receive health care services

admission, clinic outpatient formal acceptance by a hospital of a patient who is to receive diagnostic services or treatment in a formally organized unit of a medical or surgical specialty or subspecialty, but who is not to be lodged in the hospital's inpatient unit

admission, emergency outpatient formal acceptance by a hospital outpatient department of a patient whose condition requires prompt attention or treatment

admission, inpatient formal acceptance by a hospital of a patient who is to receive health care services while lodged in an area of the hospital reserved for continuous nursing services

admission, newborn inpatient formal acceptance by a hospital of a patient newly born in the hospital

admission, outpatient formal acceptance by a hospital of a patient who is to receive health care services but who is not to be lodged in an area of the hospital for continuous nursing services

admission, preadmission process for formal acceptance by a hospital of a patient for preliminary tests on an outpatient basis prior to admission as an inpatient

admission, referred outpatient formal acceptance by a hospital of an outpatient who, upon the referral of a physician or another hospital, is to receive only designated services

admissions review See *review, admissions*

admitting manager See *admitting officer*

admitting officer person who arranges for admission and discharge of patients and directs the activities of the admitting department

adult day care provision during the day, on a regular basis, of a range of services, which may include health, medical, psychological, social, nutritional, and educational services, that allow a person to function in the home environment

adult day health services provision during the day of medical or other health-related services to patients who are ambulatory or who can be transported and whose physical or mental condition does not require continuous care

affiliated hospital See *hospital, affiliated*

alcoholism rehabilitation center facility with an organized professional and trained staff that provides treatment and rehabilitative services to alcoholic patients

alcoholism treatment service service providing diagnosis and treatment of alcoholic patients

allergist physician who specializes in the diagnosis and treatment of allergies

allowable cost See *cost, allowable*

ambulance attendant See *emergency medical technician*

ambulatory care provision of health care services to outpatients and to other patients who do not require admission to the hospital as inpatients

ambulatory care center facility with an organized professional staff that provides various medical and health-related services to patients who do not require admission to a hospital as inpatients

ambulatory surgery service service providing surgery for patients who are admitted and discharged on the day of surgery

ambulatory surgical facility freestanding or hospital-based facility, with an organized professional staff, that provides surgical services to patients who do not require an inpatient bed

ancillary services those services other than room, board, and medical and nursing services, such as laboratory, radiology, pharmacy, and therapy services, that are provided to hospital patients in the course of care

anesthesiologist physician who specializes in the administration of local or general anesthesia before and during surgery, performs cardiac and respiratory resuscitation, and alleviates chronic pain through anesthesia treatments

anesthesiologist assistant person who, only under the direct supervision of a physician or dentist, assists in the administration of anesthetics

anesthesiology service service providing administration of anesthetics to patients undergoing surgery and anesthesia treatment for cardiac and respiratory resuscitation and alleviation of chronic pain

anesthetist physician or registered nurse who administers anesthetic agents to patients before and after surgical and obstetrical operations and other medical and dental procedures See also *anesthesiologist* and *nurse anesthetist*

animal care technologist person who cares for animals used in laboratory experiments, biological tests, and medical research

attending physician See *physician, attending*

audiologist person qualified by a master's degree in audiology who evaluates and treats patients with impaired hearing

audiology service service providing diagnosis and treatment for patients with impaired hearing

audiometrician person who administers hearing tests prescribed by audiologists and physicians to patients for diagnostic and evaluative purposes

audit, medical retrospective review by medical staff members of selected hospital medical records, performed for the purpose of evaluating the quality and quantity of medical care in relation to accepted standards

audit, patient care retrospective review by a multidisciplinary professional committee of selected hospital medical records, performed for the purpose of evaluating the quality and quantity of care provided in relation to accepted standards

authenticate denote authorship of an entry made in a patient's medical record by means of a written signature, identifiable initials, a computer key, or a personally used rubber stamp

autopsy, hospital postmortem examination performed by a pathologist or other member of the medical staff on the body of a person who had at some time been a patient of the hospital

autopsy rate, adjusted number of autopsies performed on patients over a given period in relation to total number of inpatient and outpatient deaths, less those bodies unavailable for autopsy

autopsy rate, gross number of autopsies performed on inpatients over a given period in relation to total number of inpatient deaths, usually expressed as the number of autopsies performed per 100 deaths

autopsy rate, net number of autopsies performed on inpatients over a given period in relation to total number of inpatient deaths, less those bodies unavailable for autopsy

auxilian member of a hospital auxiliary who may or may not be an in-service volunteer within the affiliated hospital See also *auxiliary, hospital*

auxiliary, hospital self-governing membership organization founded by persons from the community to assist the hospital in promoting the health and welfare of the community

Bb

bacteriologist physician, medical technologist, or other qualified person who specializes in the study of bacteria for clinical or research purposes

bassinet See *bed, newborn*

bed, adult inpatient hospital bed regularly maintained for adult inpatients who are receiving continuing hospital services

bed, day hospital bed regularly maintained for use during the day by patients who require partial hospitalization

bed, hospital accommodation including lodging, food, and routine medical and nursing services provided in a hospital for care of patients See also *bed, inpatient*

bed, incubator hospital bed regularly maintained for premature and other infants who require special environmental conditions

bed, inpatient hospital bed regularly maintained for use by inpatients

bed, isolation hospital bed regularly maintained for inpatients who require isolation

bed, newborn hospital bed regularly maintained for infants newly born in the hospital

bed, night hospital bed regularly maintained for use during the night by patients who require partial hospitalization

bed, occupied hospital bed assigned to designated inpatients

bed, outpatient hospital bed regularly maintained for patients who require medical services for less than 24 hours

bed, partial hospitalization See *bed, day; bed, night*

bed, pediatric See *bed, pediatric inpatient*

bed, pediatric inpatient hospital bed regularly maintained for pediatric inpatients, other than newborns, who are receiving continuing hospital services

bed, resident bed regularly maintained in a residential care facility for use by persons who require custodial and personal services but not nursing or medical services

bed, specialty bed regularly maintained for a specific category of patients

bed, swing hospital bed regularly maintained for both short-term and long-term use depending on need

bed, temporary hospital bed provided for use by patients at times when the patient census exceeds the number of beds regularly maintained

bed capacity See *beds, constructed; beds, licensed; beds, regularly maintained*

bed count number of beds regularly maintained by a hospital for inpatients

bed count, adult inpatient number of beds regularly maintained by a hospital for adult inpatients

bed count, child inpatient number of beds regularly maintained by a hospital for pediatric inpatients

bed count, newborn number of beds regularly maintained by a hospital for infants newly born in the hospital

bed size See *bed count*

bed turnover rate average number of times over a given period that there is a change of occupant of a bed regularly maintained by a hospital

beds, constructed number of beds that a hospital can accommodate

beds, licensed number of beds that a hospital is licensed or certified by the state to maintain

beds, regularly maintained number of beds that a hospital has regularly set up and staffed for use

biochemist person who specializes in the study of biochemical compounds for clinical or research purposes

bioengineer person who applies engineering and technological concepts to improve the understanding of biological and anatomical systems

biomedical engineer person who applies the principles of engineering and the physical sciences to solving problems related to biology and medicine

biomedical engineering field of study that combines knowledge of engineering with the disciplines of medicine, biology, and physiology to develop technological devices for improving health care

biomedical engineering department department providing biomedical engineering services

biomedical engineering technician See *biomedical equipment technician*

biomedical equipment technician person who operates, maintains, and repairs biomedical equipment

biomedical laboratory technician See *biomedical equipment technician*

birthing room in-hospital combination labor and delivery unit with a homelike setting, for mothers and fathers who have completed specified childbirth courses and wish to jointly participate in the birth

birth room See *birthing room*

blood, outdated donated whole blood that has been stored under refrigeration for more than 21 days and therefore is unusable for transfusion

blood, unprocessed whole donated blood that has been drawn into a container but has not been serologically tested, grouped, or typed

blood bank facility for the procurement, drawing, processing, storage, and distribution of whole blood and its components

blood bank, commercial blood bank whose surplus income inures to the benefit of the owner(s)

blood bank, community not-for-profit blood bank serving various hospitals in a community

blood bank, hospital blood bank owned and operated by a hospital primarily to meet the needs of its own patients

blood bank, proprietary See *blood bank, commercial*

blood bank technologist certified medical technologist or other qualified person, both qualified by an accredited medical technology program, who, under the supervision of a pathologist, a physician, or qualified scientist, collects blood and its components from donors and stores, prepares, and processes it for use in transfusions See also *medical technologist; medical technologist, certified*

blood banking procurement, drawing, processing, storage, and distribution of blood and its components

blood distribution issue, exchange, or sale by a blood bank of processed whole blood or blood components and derivatives

blood processing serological testing, grouping, and typing of whole blood for direct use and preparation of blood components and derivatives

blood replacement deposit fee payable by the recipient of blood or blood components in lieu of replacing the blood or components received See also *donor, replacement blood*

blood repository facility for storage and distribution of both whole blood and its components by arrangement with a blood bank

board certified term that describes a physician or other health professional who has passed an examination given by a medical specialty board and has been certified by that board as a specialist in that subject

board-designated funds See *funds, board-designated*

board eligible term that describes a physician or other health professional who is eligible for specialty board examination on the basis of such requirements as graduation from an approved school, training experience of specified type and length, and specified time in practice or on the job

board of directors See *governing body*

board of governors See *governing body*

board of trustees See *governing body*

boarder person other than a patient, physician, or staff member, such as a parent or spouse of an inpatient, who is temporarily housed in a hospital

buildings and grounds, director of See *engineer, administrative*

burn care unit intensive care unit for treatment of inpatients with severe burns

Cc

cancer registry See *tumor registry*

capital expenditure review See *review, capital expenditure*

capitation method of payment for health services in which an individual or institutional provider is paid a fixed, per capita amount for each person served without regard to the actual number or nature of services provided

captive insurance company insurance company owned and operated directly or indirectly by one or more corporations for the sole purpose of protecting the corporation's assets by insuring the owners against loss

cardiac care nurse See *nurse, cardiac care*

cardiac care unit intensive care unit for treatment and continuous monitoring of inpatients with acute or impending cardiac disorders

cardiac catheterization service service providing for examination of the circulatory system by means of catheterization through a vein or artery into the heart

cardiac surveillance unit See *cardiac care unit*

cardiologist physician who specializes in the diagnosis and treatment of cardiovascular diseases

cardiology service service providing diagnosis and treatment of patients with cardiovascular disorders

cardiovascular technician person who operates equipment used in making X rays, x-ray movies, and closed-circuit telecasts of the vascular and circulatory systems

care plan formal written plan of activities to be conducted by personnel of a long-term care facility, home health agency, hospital, or other health facility on behalf of a patient and to be used to evaluate that patient's needs and progress See also *nursing care plan*

carrier insurance company, prepayment plan, or government agency that, under a health insurance or prepayment program, administers claims submitted for or by its beneficiaries and, in certain cases, directly provides services See also *intermediary*

case mix grouping of patients possessing similar clinical attributes and output utilization patterns, primarily for purposes of cost accounting and reimbursement

CAT computed axial tomography See also *computed tomography service*

catastrophic insurance See *insurance, catastrophic*

catchment area geographic area defined and served by a hospital and delineated on the basis of such factors as population distribution, natural geographic boundaries, and transportation accessibility

CCU See *cardiac care unit*

census, average daily average number of inpatients, excluding newborns, receiving care each day during a reported period

census, boarder number of boarders in a hospital at a given time

census, inpatient number of inpatients in a hospital at a given time

central service department department providing for sterilization, storage, and distribution of sterile equipment and supplies

central service technician person who sterilizes, maintains, and inventories medical and surgical instruments and other hospital supplies

certificate of need certificate of approval issued usually by a state health planning agency to health care facilities that propose to construct or modify a health care facility, incur a major capital expenditure, or offer a new or different health service

certification process of evaluation and formal recognition that a person, device, or facility meets the standards of a certifying organization

certified formally recognized by a certifying organization as meeting its standards

certified hospital See *hospital, certified*

certified registered nurse anesthetist See *nurse anesthetist, certified registered*

chain organization See *multihospital system*

chairman of service See *chief of service*

chaplain member of the clergy who provides pastoral counseling to patients and their families and to hospital staff

chaplaincy service service administering religious activities and providing pastoral counseling to patients and their families and to hospital staff

charge dollar amount charged by a hospital, physician, or other health care provider for a unit of service, such as a day's stay in an inpatient unit or a specific medical procedure

charge nurse See *nurse, charge*

charge, covered charge for services provided to an insured patient that is recognized as payable by a third-party payer

charge, daily service dollar amount charged by a hospital for a day's stay in an inpatient care unit

charity allowance reduced charge for health care service in recognition of a patient's indigence or medical indigence

chemical-dependency service service providing diagnosis and treatment of drug-dependent patients

chemistry technologist medical technologist who conducts chemical analyses of body fluids and exudates See also *medical technologist*

chief engineer See *engineer, chief*

chief executive officer person usually qualified by a master's degree in an accredited educational program in health services or business administration who is appointed by the hospital governing body and who directs the overall management of the hospital

chief financial officer person who is responsible for a hospital's fiscal integrity and for planning, organizing, and controlling all financial operations

chief of service member of a hospital medical staff who is elected or appointed to serve as the medical and administrative head of a clinical department

chief of staff member of a hospital medical staff who is elected, appointed, or employed by the hospital and who serves as the medical and administrative head of the medical staff

childbirth center freestanding or hospital-based facility that provides prenatal, childbirth, and postnatal care, often incorporating family-centered maternity care concepts and practices

chiropractor person qualified by a postsecondary program in chiropractic and licensed by the state who treats disease primarily by adjustment of parts of the body, especially the spinal column

chronic disease hospital See *hospital, chronic disease*

circulating nurse See *nurse, circulating*

circulation technologist See *perfusion technologist*

city hospital See *hospital, municipal*

claims-made policy form of liability insurance that protects the insured against any claims made against the insured for the limited period (usually one year) during which the policy is in effect See also *professional liability insurance*

claims review See *review, claims*

clinic See *outpatient service*

clinic clerk person who performs routine clerical and reception tasks in a hospital clinic or outpatient department or a freestanding ambulatory care facility

clinical chemist person who specializes in the study of chemical compounds for clinical or research purposes

clinical clerk student of a medical or dental school who, as part of the school's curriculum, receives clinical experience by performing specific supervised duties in a hospital See also *clinical clerkship*

clinical clerkship undergraduate clinical experience provided to a student of a hospital-affiliated medical or dental school as part of the school's curriculum

clinical engineer See *engineer, clinical*

clinical engineering department department providing maintenance and repair of medical devices

clinical instructor, nurse See *nurse clinical instructor*

clinical laboratory laboratory for examination of material derived from the human body by means of bacteriological, biochemical, cytologic, hematologic, histologic, and serologic tests

clinical nurse specialist See *nurse specialist, clinical*

clinical privileges See *privileges, clinical*

clinical psychologist See *psychologist, clinical*

clinical psychology service service providing counseling of and psychometric services to patients with mental or emotional problems

COB See *coordination of benefits*

cobalt therapy service service providing radioactive cobalt therapy for patients with malignancies

coinsurance requirement of an insurance policy or prepayment plan that a predetermined portion or percentage of the provider's charges be paid by the beneficiary

community health center organization capable of delivering both health care and related social services, generally in a geographic area with scarce or nonexistent health services

community hospital See *hospital, community*

community living facility See *halfway house*

community mental health center organization capable of delivering mental health services to individuals who reside or are employed in a defined geographic area

community relations director See *public relations, director of*

community residential facility facility that provides living accommodations and guidance in daily living activities principally to mentally retarded persons See also *intermediate care facility for the mentally retarded*

comprehensive health care services that meet the total health care needs of a patient

comprehensive health care delivery system health care facilities and professionals organized and coordinated to provide comprehensive health care to a defined population group

comprehensive health planning process of using data analysis to plan maximum efficiency in the use of environmental, occupational health, and health education resources for a given population

comprehensive health planning agency agency originally established under the Comprehensive Health Planning and Public Health Services Amendments of 1966 (Public Law 89-749) to perform specified health care planning functions, later superseded by the health systems agencies, state health planning and development agencies, and statewide health coordinating councils established by the Health Planning and Resources Development Act of 1974 (Public Law 93-641)

comptroller See *controller*

computed axial tomography See *computed tomography service*

computed tomography service service providing diagnosis of disease through visualization of internal body structures by means of computer synthesis of x-ray particles

concurrent review See *review, concurrent*

consent See *informed consent*

consolidation formal combination of two or more hospitals into a single new legal entity that has an identity separate from any of the preexisting hospitals See also *merger*

consortium voluntary alliance of institutions for a specific purpose and usually located in the same geographic area

consultant, hospital person who, as an independent contractor, provides advice on organization and management to hospitals

consultant, medical physician who, at the request of an attending physician, provides professional service to or advice regarding a patient of the attending physician

continued-stay review See *review, continued-stay*

contract physician See *physician, contract*

contract service service rendered to or on behalf of a hospital under contract with an organization or person

contractual adjustment bookkeeping adjustment to reflect uncollectible differences between established charges for services rendered to insured persons and rates payable for those services under contracts with third-party payers

controller person who directs a hospital's day-to-day financial administration, accounting, business services, financial and statistical reporting, and related activities and who may serve as the chief financial officer

coordination of benefits claims review procedure by which a claim covered by two or more carriers is identified and the liability of each determined for the purpose of avoiding duplication of payments

copayment specified share of total liability for which the insured is responsible; for example, a specific amount per hospital day or a percentage of the total bill

coronary care unit See *cardiac care unit*

cost expense incurred in providing services

cost, allowable cost incurred by a provider in the course of providing service that is recognized as payable by a third-party payer

cost-based reimbursement See *reimbursement, cost-based*

county hospital See *hospital, county*

covered charge See *charge, covered*

credentialing generic term referring to the processes of certification and licensure of health care personnel and the formal recognition of professional or technical competence

critical care nurse See *nurse, critical care*

critical care physician See *physician, critical care*

critical care unit See *intensive care unit*

CT See *computed tomography service*

custodial care provision of board, room, and other nonmedical personal assistance, generally on a long-term basis

custodial care facility See *residential care facility*

cytologist physician or medical technologist who specializes in the study of cellular changes in the body as a result of disease, especially cancer See also *cytopathologist* and *cytotechnologist*

cytology laboratory laboratory for microscopic examination of human cells, especially cancer

cytopathologist pathologist who specializes in the study of cellular changes in the body as a result of disease, especially cancer

cytotechnologist medical technologist who specializes in laboratory evaluation of cellular changes in the body as a result of disease, especially cancer See also *medical technologist*

Dd

daily service charge See *charge, daily service*

day, charity care services and accommodations provided by a hospital to one inpatient over one 24-hour period for which the hospital waives payment

day, inpatient bed count number of inpatient beds available for use in one 24-hour period

day, inpatient service services and accommodations provided by a hospital to one inpatient over one 24-hour period See also *day equivalents, inpatient*

day, occupied bed period of service between the census-taking hours on two successive calendar days, the day of discharge being counted only when the patient was admitted the same day

day, partial hospitalization services and accommodations provided to one patient in a partial hospitalization program in one 24-hour period

day, patient See *day, inpatient service*

day, resident services and accommodations provided by a residential care facility to one patient in one 24-hour period

day bed See *bed, day*

day care See *adult day care*

day equivalents, inpatient sum of all inpatient service days, plus, over the same period, the estimated volume of outpatient services expressed in units equivalent to inpatient service days

day health care services provision during the day, generally in hospitals, nursing homes, or facilities specifically designated as adult day health care facilities, of medical and health-related services to patients who are ambulatory or can be transported and who regularly require such services for a substantial number of daytime hours but do not require continuous inpatient care

days, adjusted inpatient service See *day equivalents, inpatient*

DDS doctor of dental science or surgery See also *dentist*

death rate, disease-specific number of deaths caused by a disease in relation to a given population over a given period, usually expressed as the number of deaths per 100,000 persons

death rate, fetal number of fetal deaths in relation to total births, that is, live births and fetal deaths combined, usually expressed as the number of early fetal deaths per 1,000 total births

death rate, hospital number of deaths of inpatients in relation to total number of inpatients over a given period

death rate, hospital infant See *death rate, hospital neonatal*

death rate, hospital maternal number of deaths of obstetric patients in a hospital in relation to total number of obstetric patients who were discharged or who died over a given period

death rate, hospital neonatal number of neonatal deaths in a hospital in relation to total number of infants born who were discharged or who died over a given period

death rate, infant number of infant deaths in relation to total number of infants born in a given population over a given period, usually expressed as the number of deaths per 1,000 live births See also *death, infant; death rate, hospital neonatal*

death rate, maternal number of deaths attributed to obstetric causes in relation to a given population of women whose pregnancies terminate over a given period, usually expressed as the number of deaths per 10,000 live births

death rate, neonatal number of neonatal deaths in relation to all infants born in a given population over a given period, usually expressed as the number of neonatal deaths per 100 or 1,000 live births

death rate, perinatal number of perinatal deaths in relation to all live births and stillbirths in a given population in a given period, usually expressed as the number of perinatal deaths per 1,000 total births

death rate, total number of deaths in relation to a given population over a given period, usually expressed as the number of deaths per 1,000 persons

deemed status status conferred on a hospital by the area professional standards review organization in formal recognition that the hospital's admissions review, continued-stay review, and medical care evaluation programs meet the PSRO's effectiveness criteria and therefore whose determinations regarding which services to Medicare, Medicaid, and Maternal and Child Health patients are appropriate for payment are regarded as final by those programs

delivery room unit for obstetric delivery and infant resuscitation

dental assistant person who directly assists a dentist in providing care to patients by performing a range of duties regulated by the Dental Practice Acts and the decisions of the dentist

dental hygienist person who, under the supervision of a dentist, assumes delegated responsibility for providing preventive and therapeutic dental services for patients

dental laboratory technician person who makes a variety of dental prostheses and appliances following the specifications described in dentists' work authorizations

dental service service providing preventive care, diagnosis, and treatment of patients to promote, maintain, or restore dental health

dental technician See *dental laboratory technician*

dentist person qualified by a doctorate in dental surgery or dental medicine and licensed by the state to practice dentistry

dermatologist physician who specializes in the diagnosis and treatment of skin disorders

detoxification service service providing treatment to diminish or remove from the body the poisonous effects of chemical substances such as alcohol or drugs, usually as the first step in the treatment of chemical-dependent patients See also *alcoholism treatment service, chemical-dependency service*

development, director of person who plans and directs a hospital's fund-raising activities

diagnosis-related group grouping of direct patient cost data determined by the diagnosis, treatment, and age of a patient, commonly referred to as DRG

diagnostic services services related to diagnosis performed by physicians, nurses, and other professional and technical personnel under the direction of a physician

diener person who maintains hospital morgue equipment and facilities and, under the supervision of a pathologist, assists in performing autopsies

diet, modified dietary regimen altered in regard to such factors as nutrients, calorie value, food content, texture, or consistency to meet special nutritional requirements of a patient

dietary department See *food service department*

dietetic assistant person qualified by a dietetic assistant program approved by the American Dietetic Association who, under the supervision of a dietetic technician, a dietitian, or an administrator and a consultant dietitian, assists in providing food service supervision and nutritional care services

dietetic technician person qualified by an associate degree program approved by the American Dietetic Association who, under the supervision of a dietitian or of an administrator and a consultant dietitian, assists in providing food service management or nutritional care services

dietitian person who meets all requirements for active membership in the American Dietetic Association and who is a specialist educated for a profession responsible for the nutritional care of individuals and groups

dietitian, administrative registered dietitian who affects the nutritional care of groups through the management of food service systems that provide optimal nutrition and high-quality food

dietitian, clinical registered dietitian who assesses nutritional needs of patients, develops and implements nutritional care plans, and evaluates and reports results appropriately

dietitian, consultant registered dietitian qualified by experience in administrative or clinical dietetic practice who provides counsel or supervision of dietary activities See also *dietitian, registered*

dietitian, registered dietitian who is registered by the Commission on Dietetic Registration upon successful completion of an examination and maintenance of continuing education requirements See also *dietitian*

dietitian, research registered dietitian qualified by advanced preparation in dietetics and research techniques who plans, investigates, interprets, evaluates, and applies knowledge in one or more phases of dietetics See also *dietitian, registered*

dietitian, teaching registered dietitian qualified by advanced preparation in dietetics or education who plans, conducts, and evaluates educational programs in dietetics See also *dietitian, registered*

diploma, nursing diploma conferred by a hospital-sponsored school of nursing, usually upon completion of a three-year program of study

director See *trustee*

disaster plan See *disaster preparedness plan*

disaster preparedness plan formal written plan of action for coordinating the response of a hospital staff in the event of a disaster within the hospital or the community

discharge, inpatient formal release by a hospital, upon a physician's direction, of an inpatient who no longer requires hospital care

discharge, outpatient formal release by a hospital, upon a physician's direction, of an outpatient who no longer requires hospital care

discharge abstract items of information, available from the medical records of patients discharged from the hospital, that are extracted and recorded in a uniform manner to provide data for statistical, reporting, research, and other purposes

discharge coordinator person who arranges with health or community agencies and institutions to engage in the care of patients upon discharge from a hospital

discharge planning centralized, coordinated program developed by a hospital to ensure that each patient has a planned program for needed continuing or follow-up care

11

discharge summary clinical resumé prepared by the physician or dentist at the conclusion of a patient's hospital stay that summarizes the chief complaint, diagnostic findings, therapy, response to treatment, and recommendations on discharge

discharge transfer See *transfer, discharge*

district hospital See *hospital, district*

donated services services provided by personnel who receive partial or no compensation

donor person who serves as a source of biological material, such as blood or an organ, or person or organization that provides a monetary gift, for example, to a hospital

donor, blood person who permits blood to be withdrawn from his or her body for medical use

donor, organ person who permits an organ to be removed from his or her body for transplantation to another person

donor, replacement blood blood donor whose donation replaces blood used by a specific patient and thereby cancels charges to the patient for blood

donor, voluntary blood blood donor who does not receive payment

DRG See *diagnosis-related group*

drug administration in hospitals, the giving by a registered nurse or other authorized person of a single dose of a drug to a patient

drug dispensing in hospitals, that part of the drug distribution process involving the preparation, packaging, labeling, record keeping, and subsequent transfer of one or more doses of a prescription drug to a patient or an intermediary (for example, nurse) for administration

drug prescription See *prescription, drug*

Ee

ECF extended care facility See also *skilled nursing facility*

ECU extended care unit See also *skilled nursing unit*

education, director of person who directs employee orientation, on-the-job training, and continuing education and, in some instances, patient community education programs

education, in-service educational activities provided to employees, including orientation, on-the-job training, and continuing education

education coordinator, in-service See *education, director of*

education department department providing staff educational programs, including orientation, on-the-job training, and continuing education and, in some instances, patient and community education programs

electroencephalographic technician person who maintains and operates electroencephalograph machines

electroencephalographic technologist person who supervises electroencephalographic technicians and, in some instances, manages an electroencephalographic laboratory

emergency situation that requires immediate intervention to assist person with potentially disabling or life-threatening conditions

emergency department physician See *physician, emergency department*

emergency medical services system system of personnel, facilities, and equipment administered by a public or not-for-profit organization delivering emergency medical services within a designated geographic area

emergency medical technician person who, under the direction of a physician, administers basic initial emergency care to patients

emergency medical technician-advanced emergency medical technician who, under the direction of a physician, administers certain emergency medical services that require intervention within the patient's body See also *emergency medical technician*

emergency medical technician-paramedic emergency medical technician who, under the supervision of a physician, administers advanced emergency medical services See also *emergency medical technician*

emergency service, hospital service providing immediate initial evaluation and treatment of acutely ill or injured patients on a 24-hour-a-day basis

employee health service service providing preemployment medical screening and health care services to employees

EMT See *emergency medical technician*

encounter instance of direct contact between a patient and a professional hospital staff member responsible for assessing and treating the condition of the patient or providing social work services

endostomy therapist See *enterostomal therapist*

endowment fund See *fund, endowment*

engineer, administrative hospital engineer who has overall administrative responsibility for planning, managing, and maintaining a hospital's physical environment, equipment, and systems

engineer, chief hospital engineer who directs and administers a hospital's equipment, buildings and grounds maintenance, and repair programs See also *engineer, administrative*

engineer, clinical person who adapts, maintains, and improves the safe use of equipment and instruments in hospitals

engineer, hospital person who is responsible for the operation of a hospital's physical plant and equipment

engineer, industrial person who uses the techniques of human and material resources management to help a hospital manage its resources

engineer, plant See *engineer, chief*

engineering and maintenance department department providing for maintenance of the hospital's physical plant, including heating, ventilating, and air-conditioning systems, utilities, telecommunications, and clinical engineering equipment

ENT specialist ear, nose, and throat specialist See also *otolaryngologist*

enterostomal therapist registered nurse qualified by an accredited program in enterostomal therapy who provides wound drainage services to patients

environmental services services such as housekeeping, laundry, maintenance, and liquid and solid waste control performed to ensure safe, sanitary, and efficient hospital operation

environmental services department department providing for maintenance of a safe and sanitary hospital through such means as control of solid and liquid wastes, radiation exposure, and pathogenic organisms See also *housekeeping department*

epidemiologist physician or other qualified person who studies the incidence, prevalence, spread, prevention, and control of disease in a community, medical facility, or specific population

epidemiologist, hospital physician, often a medical epidemiologist, or other qualified person who has responsibility for direction of a hospital's infection control program

epidemiologist, medical physician who studies and predicts the occurrence of disease in a community or other specific population

epidemiologist, nurse registered nurse, usually with postgraduate training in epidemiology, who studies the incidence of communicable disease in the community

epidemiology department See *infection control committee*

episode of hospital care measure of the services provided in a continuous course of care by a hospital to a patient for a particular medical problem or condition, such as sequence of emergency, inpatient, and outpatient services

executive director See *chief executive officer*

executive vice-president See *chief executive officer*

extended care See *skilled nursing care*

extended care facility See *skilled nursing facility*

extended care unit unit for treatment of inpatients who require convalescent, rehabilitative, or long-term skilled nursing care See also *skilled nursing unit*

extern medical or dental student who, as an extracurricular activity under professional supervision in the hospital, provides medical or dental care to patients and who receives payment for services

extracorporeal technician See *perfusion technologist*

Ff

family-centered maternity/newborn care delivery of safe, high-quality health care while recognizing, focusing on, and adapting to both the physical and psychosocial needs of the client-patient, the family, and the newly born

family planning service service providing family planning assistance to patients

family practice service service providing general medical care to members of family groups, regardless of age

family practitioner physician who assumes continuing responsibility for supervising the health and coordinating the care of all members of a family, regardless of age

federal government hospital See *hospital, federal government*

financial director See *chief financial officer*

first-dollar coverage insurance or prepayment coverage under which the third-party payer assumes liability for covered services as soon as the first dollar of expense for such services is incurred, without requiring the insured to pay a deductible

float nurse See *nurse, float*

float pool group of nurses available for assignment to duty on an ad hoc basis, usually to assist in times of unusually heavy work loads or to assume the duties of absent nursing personnel

FMC See *foundation for medical care*

food service administrator person who plans and manages a food service system

food service department department providing for food preparation and services to patients and hospital personnel and also providing nutritional care to patients

for-profit hospital See *hospital, investor-owned*

foundation for medical care not-for-profit organization, usually of physicians and usually sponsored by a local or state medical society, that contracts with government and private health insurers to provide medical services to a designated population at a predetermined cost and/or to perform various utilization review activities

fund, endowment account that is established by a donor and whose revenue may be spent for a specified purpose or for use at the discretion of a hospital governing board but whose principal must be maintained in perpetuity

fund, general money used at the discretion of the administration and the governing board in the regular operation of a hospital

fund, permanent See *fund, endowment*

fund, specific-purpose account that is established by a donor and whose principal and income are used solely for a designated purpose

funds, board-designated money set aside by a hospital governing board for a specified purpose

funds, restricted money donated to a hospital that can be expended for a specified purpose only

funds, unrestricted money donated to a hospital that can be expended at the discretion of the administration or the governing board

Gg

gastroenterologist physician who specializes in the diagnosis and treatment of diseases of the digestive system

general-duty nurse See *nurse, staff*

general fund See *fund, general*

general hospital See *hospital, general*

general practitioner See *family practitioner*

genetic counseling service service providing counseling to prospective parents concerning the potential for genetic defects in their offspring

geriatrician physician who specializes in the diagnosis and treatment of diseases of the aging and the aged

governing board See *governing body*

governing body group, board, agency, or corporation that has ultimate responsibility and authority for a hospital's organizational policies, administration, and quality of care

group practice combined practice of three or more physicians and/or dentists who share office space, equipment, records, office personnel, expenses, and income

group practice, multispecialty physician and/or dentist group practice in which at least one physician is a family practitioner, internist, or general surgeon and the others practice other specialties

group practice, prepaid multispecialty group practice in which services are provided to an enrolled population on a prepayment basis

group practice, single-specialty physician and/or dentist group practice in which all practice the same specialty

gynecologist physician who specializes in the diseases and disorders of the female reproductive organs and functions

Hh

halfway house facility with a staff that provides guidance, treatment, and rehabilitative services to patients who require continuing treatment of mental illness, alcoholism, or drug abuse but do not require inpatient care

head nurse See *nurse, head*

health care provision by professional and paraprofessional personnel of services for the maintenance of health, prevention of illness, and treatment of illness or injury

health care delivery See *comprehensive health care delivery system*

health care institution institution with permanent facilities and staff that provides medical and/or health-related services

health economics social science that studies the demand for and supply of health care resources and the impact of health services on the health of a population

health economist social scientist who conducts research and analytical studies pertaining to the allocation of health care resources

health educator person who is responsible for the development and/or implementation of health education programs

health facility licensing agency, state unit of state government legally empowered to set standards for and grant permission to operate health care institutions

health maintenance preservation of the physical, mental, and social well-being of a person

health maintenance organization organization that has management responsibility for providing comprehensive health care services on a prepayment basis to voluntarily enrolled persons within a designated population

health physicist physicist who directs research, training, and monitoring programs to protect patients and laboratory personnel from radiation hazards and who sometimes computes the dosage and treatment plan for radiation therapy

health planner person, usually employed by a planning agency, hospital, or other health care facility, who is responsible for planning for the health needs of an area, population, type of health service, or health program

health planning planning concerned with improving health, whether undertaken for an area, population, type of health service, or health program

health planning agency See *health systems agency; state health planning and development agency*

health promotion process of fostering awareness, influencing attitudes, and identifying alternatives so that individuals can make informed choices and change their behavior in order to achieve an optimum level of physical and mental health

health-related care institution institution with permanent facilities, including inpatient or resident beds, and staff that provides health-related services that may include limited nursing services

health-related services services other than the provision of medical care that directly or indirectly contribute to the physical or mental health and well-being of patients, such as protective, personal, and social services

health service area geographic area designated under the Health Planning and Resources Development Act of 1974 (Public Law 93-641), on the basis of such factors as geography, political boundaries, population, and health resources, for the effective planning and development of health services

health services services that directly or indirectly contribute to the health and well-being of patients, such as medical, nursing, and other health-related services

health systems agency not-for-profit organization or unit of local government designated under the Health Planning and Resources Development Act of 1974 (Public Law 93-641) to perform various health planning functions within a defined geographic area, develop the areawide health systems plan, conduct certificate-of-need reviews, and review the proposed use of some federal health funds See also *health systems plan*

health systems analyst systems analyst who uses the techniques of human and material resources management to help a hospital manage its resources

health systems plan five-year plan prepared by a health systems agency for its health service area specifying the health goals and objectives considered appropriate for the area See also *health systems agency*

hematologist physician or other qualified person who specializes in the diagnosis and treatment of disease of the blood and bone marrow

hematology laboratory laboratory for examination of blood specimens by means of serologic and other tests

hematology technologist medical technologist who specializes in the performance of blood tests for use by physicians in the diagnosis and treatment of disease of the blood and bone marrow See also *medical technologist*

hemodialysis technician registered nurse who operates an artificial kidney machine in treating patients with kidney disorders

hemodialysis unit unit for treatment of patients with renal insufficiency by means of hemodialysis

high-risk nursery See *neonatal intensive care unit*

Hill-Burton program federal program of financial assistance created by the Hospital Survey and Construction Act of 1946 for the construction and modernization of health care facilities

histologic technician medical laboratory technician who specializes in the preparation of tissue specimens for microscopic examination See also *medical laboratory technician*

histologic technologist medical technologist who specializes in the preparation and study of human tissue specimens See also *medical technologist*

histologist pathologist, biologist, or laboratory technologist who specializes in the examination and study of cells and tissues

histopathologist physician who specializes in the study of minute changes in
diseased tissue

histopathology laboratory laboratory
for microscopic examination of tissue
specimens

HMO See *health maintenance
organization*

holistic health health as viewed from the
perspective that the patient is collec-
tively more than the sum of his or her
parts—that body, mind, and spirit must
be in harmony to achieve optimum
health—and that therefore a multidisciplinary approach to health care is
required

home care program organizational
entity that provides home health services in the patient's home See also
home health care

home care program, hospital-based
home care program sponsored by a
hospital

home care service See *home health
agency*

home for the aged residential care facility that provides services, such as
health-related, personal, social, or
recreational services, to aged persons

home health agency public or private
organization that provides, either
directly or through arrangements with
other organizations, home health services in the patient's home

home health aide person who, under the
supervision of a home health or welfare
agency, assists elderly, ill, or disabled
persons with household chores,
bathing, and other daily living needs
See also *homemaker*

home health care provision of health
services such as nursing, therapy, and
health-related homemaker or social
services in the patient's home

home health care, intensive home
health care provided to persons with
serious illness whose medical condition is unstable and who require con-
centrated physician and nursing
management

home health care, intermediate home
health care provided to persons whose
medical condition is not expected to
fluctuate significantly as rehabilitation
is achieved or the disease progresses

home health care, maintenance home
health care provided to persons whose
primary needs are usually for personal
care and/or other supportive environmental and social services

home health services See *home health
care*

homemaker person who, under the
supervision of a home health or welfare
agency, assists elderly, ill, or disabled
persons with household chores, such as
cooking and cleaning See also *home
health aide*

hospice See *hospice care*

hospice care care that addresses the
physical, spiritual, emotional, psychological, social, financial, and legal needs
of the dying patient and his or her family; that is provided by an interdiscipli-
nary team of professionals and
volunteers in a variety of settings, both
inpatient and at home; and that
includes bereavement care for the
family

hospital health care institution with an
organized medical and professional
staff, and with permanent facilities that
include inpatient beds, that provides
medical, nursing, and other health-
related services to patients (each state
has its own definition of *hospital* for
accreditation purposes)

hospital, accredited hospital recognized
upon inspection by the Joint Commission on Accreditation of Hospitals as
meeting its standards for quality of care
for the safety and maintenance of the
physical plant, and for organization,
administration, and governance

hospital, acute hospital that treats
patients in an acute phase of illness or
injury

hospital, affiliated hospital that is affiliated in some degree with another institution or program, for example, a medical school, a shared services organization, a multihospital system, or a religious organization

hospital, certified hospital recognized by the U.S. Department of Health and Human Services as meeting its standards for participation as a provider in the Medicare program

hospital, chronic disease hospital that provides medical and skilled nursing services to patients with long-term illnesses who are not in an acute phase but who require an intensity of services not available in nursing homes

hospital, city See *hospital, municipal*

hospital, community hospital, usually short-term general nonfederal, whose services are available for use primarily by residents of the community in which it is located

hospital, county hospital that is controlled by an agency of county government

hospital, delegated hospital recognized by the area professional standards review organization as meeting its effectiveness criteria in performing all three required review functions—admissions review, continued-stay review, and medical care evaluation—and therefore whose determinations regarding which services to Medicare, Medicaid, and Maternal and Child Health patients are appropriate for payment are regarded as final by those programs

hospital, district hospital that is controlled by a political subdivision of a state, which subdivision is created solely for the purpose of establishing and maintaining health care institutions

hospital, federal government hospital that is managed by an agency or department of federal government

hospital, for-profit See *hospital, investor-owned*

hospital, general hospital that provides diagnostic and therapeutic services to patients for a variety of medical conditions, both surgical and nonsurgical

hospital, investor-owned hospital that is owned and operated by a corporation or an individual and that operates on a for-profit basis

hospital, licensed hospital granted by an appropriate state agency the legal right to operate in accordance with the requirements of the state

hospital, long-term hospital that treats patients who are not in an acute phase of illness

hospital, municipal hospital that is controlled by an agency of municipal government

hospital, night hospital that provides health and personal care services to patients only at night, often to those who no longer require continuous inpatient care but are not yet able to live independently

hospital, nondelegated hospital not recognized by the area professional standards review organization as meeting its effectiveness criteria in performing all three required review functions—admissions review, continued-stay review, and medical care evaluation—or hospital that elects not to perform those review functions in accordance with area PSRO requirements

hospital, nonfederal government hospital that is managed by an agency or department of state or local government

hospital, not-for-profit hospital that operates on a not-for-profit basis under the ownership and control of a private corporation

hospital, partially delegated hospital recognized by the area professional standards review organization as meeting its effectiveness criteria in performing one or two but not all three required review functions—admissions review, continued-stay review, or medical care evaluation—and therefore whose determinations regarding which services to Medicare, Medicaid, and Maternal and Child Health patients are appropriate for payment are limited accordingly by those programs

hospital, private investor-owned or not-for-profit hospital that is controlled by a legal entity other than a government agency

hospital, psychiatric hospital that provides diagnostic and treatment services to patients with mental or emotional disorders

hospital, registered hospital recognized by the American Hospital Association as having the essential specific characteristics of a hospital

hospital, rehabilitation See *rehabilitation facility*

hospital, satellite part of a hospital that is geographically separated from the hospital and that offers limited services to persons in its vicinity

hospital, security hospital controlled by, physically located within or attached to, and servicing the inmates of a penal institution

hospital, short-term hospital in which the average length of stay for all patients is less than 30 days or in which more than 50 percent of all patients are admitted to units where the average length of stay is less than 30 days

hospital, specialty hospital that provides services to patients with specified medical conditions or for special categories of patients

hospital, teaching hospital with accredited programs in medical, allied health, and/or nursing education

hospital, voluntary private hospital that is autonomous, self-established, and self-supported

hospital engineer See *engineer, hospital*

hospital epidemiologist See *epidemiologist, hospital*

house staff aggregate body of physicians and dentists in training who participate in an accredited program of graduate medical education sponsored by a hospital

housekeeper, executive housekeeping director certified by the National Executive Housekeepers' Association See also *housekeeping director*

housekeeping aide person who, under the supervision of the housekeeping supervisor, cleans and services a hospital's premises and furnishings in accordance with its housekeeping program

housekeeping department department providing for cleaning of hospital premises and furnishings, including control of pathogenic organisms

housekeeping director person who specifies and monitors the hospital's housekeeping quality standards and work procedures according to prescribed authoritative norms and manages the overall housekeeping program

housekeeping manager See *housekeeping director*

housekeeping supervisor person who oversees the day-to-day execution of the housekeeping program of a hospital

HSA See *health systems agency*

human resources developer See *education, director of*

Ii

ICF See *intermediate care facility*

ICF/MR See *intermediate care facility for the mentally retarded*

ICU See *intensive care unit*

inclusive rate See *rate, inclusive*

incubator See *bed, incubator*

incubator, isolation incubator bed regularly maintained for premature and other infants who require isolation

indigence, medical condition of having insufficient income to pay for adequate medical care without depriving oneself or dependents of food, clothing, shelter, and other essentials of living

industrial engineer See *engineer, industrial*

infection, community-acquired infection acquired by a patient in the community before admission to the hospital that may have its clinical onset when the patient is hospitalized See also *infection, nosocomial*

infection, nosocomial infection acquired during hospitalization that is neither present nor incubating at the time of hospital admission unless related to prior hospitalization and that may become clinically manifest after discharge from the hospital

infection control policies and procedures followed by a hospital to minimize the risk of infection to patients and staff

infection control committee hospital committee composed of infection control personnel and medical, nursing, laboratory, and administrative staff members (and occasionally others, such as dietary or housekeeping staff members) whose purpose is to oversee infection control activities

infection control nurse See *nurse, infection control*

information systems director person who directs and administers the operation of a hospital's data processing facilities

informed consent legal concept requiring a patient or the patient's guardian to be advised of and to understand the risks attendant to a proposed procedure or treatment, usually indicated by a signed written statement

inhalation therapist See *respiratory therapist*

inhalation therapy See *respiratory therapy*

inpatient person who receives medical, dental, or other health-related services while lodged in a hospital or other health care institution for at least one night

inpatient, adult inpatient over a certain age as determined by the hospital

inpatient, ambulatory inpatient who is able to walk about and does not require confinement to bed

inpatient, child See *inpatient, pediatric*

inpatient, pediatric inpatient under a certain age as determined by the hospital

inpatient care institution health care institution with an organized professional staff and permanent facilities, including inpatient beds, that provides medical and continuous nursing services to patients

inpatient care unit unit for treatment of inpatients, often grouped according to diagnosis or other common characteristics

inpatient care unit, mixed unit for treatment of inpatients not grouped according to diagnosis or other common characteristics

in-service education See *education, in-service*

in-service education department See *education department*

insurance, catastrophic insurance that protects the insured against all or a percentage of loss not covered by other insurance or prepayment plan or insurance in excess of specified amounts or other dollar or benefit limits or incurred under specified circumstances

insurance, major medical catastrophic insurance that protects the insured against all or a percentage of loss incurred as the result of severe or prolonged illness or disability whose costs exceed a specified dollar amount

insurance, professional liability See *professional liability insurance*

insurance clerk person who computes health insurance benefits and maintains records pertaining to such benefits

intensive care unit unit for treatment and continuous monitoring of inpatients with life-threatening conditions

intensive care unit, medical intensive care unit for nonsurgical inpatients

intensive care unit, neonatal unit for treatment and continuous monitoring of infants with life-threatening conditions who are less than 23 days old upon admission to the unit

intensive care unit, pediatric intensive care unit for pediatric inpatients

intensive care unit, surgical intensive care unit for postoperative high-risk inpatients

interim rate See *rate, interim*

intermediary Blue Cross Plan, private insurance company, or other public or private agency selected by health care providers to pay claims under Medicare

intermediate care facility facility that provides health-related services to persons with a variety of physical or emotional conditions who do not require the degree of care provided by a hospital or skilled nursing facility but who require the care and services available through institutional facilities

intermediate care facility for the mentally retarded intermediate care facility that provides care solely or particularly for the mentally retarded See also *community residential facility*

intern person with formal training in a profession who undergoes a period of practical experience, usually under the supervision of a person experienced in that profession

intern, nurse person with formal training in nursing who undergoes a period of practical clinical experience, usually under the supervision of a head nurse or designated person in the clinical area

internist physician who specializes in the diagnosis and nonsurgical treatment of disorders of the internal organ systems

intravenous team group of registered nurses and licensed practical nurses qualified by on-the-job training who, under the direction of a physician, administer intravenous therapy

investor-owned hospital See *hospital, investor-owned*

Jj

joint conference committee hospital committee, composed of governing board, administration, and medical staff members, whose purpose is to facilitate communication between the groups

joint planning development by two or more heath care provider organizations of a strategic plan to serve the health care needs of the area in which they are located and that may result in the sharing of services, either clinical or administrative, or the sharing of data and long-range plans, without any sharing of assets

joint underwriting association independent organization established, usually for a limited period, for pooling resources of various insurance carriers to provide certain liability coverage for institutions or professionals who can not obtain coverage from private insurance companies

JUA See *joint underwriting association*

Kk

kidney dialysis unit See *hemodialysis unit*

Ll

labor room hospital room regularly maintained for maternity patients who are in active labor

laboratory assistant See *medical laboratory technician*

laboratory technician See *medical laboratory technician*

laboratory technologist See *medical technologist*

laundry department department providing for laundering, storage, and distribution of linens and uniforms

laundry manager person who specifies and monitors the hospital's laundry quality standards and work procedures according to prescribed authoritative norms and coordinates the activities of the laundry department

length of stay number of calendar days that elapse between an inpatient's admission and discharge

length of stay, average average stay of all or a class of inpatients discharged over a given period, derived by dividing the number of inpatient days by the number of admissions

librarian, health sciences person qualified by graduate degree in library/information science from a program accredited by the American Library Association, or by documented equivalent training and experience, who provides library services to all hospital personnel

library, health sciences library providing for acquisition, storage, and retrieval of health sciences information materials for hospital personnel

library, hospital See *library, health sciences*

library, medical See *library, health sciences*

library, patient library providing for acquisition, storage, and retrieval of books and other materials for patients

licensed having the legal right, granted by an appropriate government agency, to practice an occupation or to engage in an activity, such as operation of a hospital

licensed hospital See *hospital, licensed*

licensed practical nurse See *nurse, licensed practical*

licensed vocational nurse See *nurse, licensed practical*

licensure process by which a government agency grants a person the legal right to practice an occupation or an organization the legal right to engage in an activity, such as operation of a hospital

lifetime reserve lifetime pool of 60 days of inpatient hospitalization benefits that may be drawn upon by a patient when he or she has exhausted the maximum benefit allowed under Medicare for a single spell of illness

living-in unit hospital room regularly maintained for mothers to assume care of newborns under the supervision of nursing personnel

long-term care provision of health, social, and/or personal care services on a recurring or continuous basis to persons with chronic physical or mental conditions who live in environments ranging from institutions to their own homes

long-term care unit See *skilled nursing unit*

long-term hospital See *hospital, chronic disease*

Mm

maintenance engineer See *engineer, chief*

major medical insurance See *insurance, major medical*

malpractice failure in providing health care services to exercise the degree of skill and care generally exercised by like professionals under similar circumstances

marketing, hospital analysis of community health care needs and institutional needs and circumstances, and subsequent planning, implementation, and evaluation of activities to meet identified needs

materials management department department providing centralized management and control of supplies and equipment from acquisition to disposition and, in many hospitals, with responsibility for central services, laundry, and print shop

materials manager person who has overall responsibility for the procurement, storage, distribution, and disposal of hospital supplies and equipment

maternity center See *childbirth center*

MD doctor of medicine See *physician*

Medicaid federal program, created by Title XIX—Medical Assistance, a 1965 amendment to the Social Security Act, administered by states, that provides health care benefits to indigent and medically indigent persons

medical assistant person who, under the direction of a physician, performs various routine administrative and nontechnical clinical tasks in a physician's office, hospital, clinic, or similar setting

medical audit See *audit, medical*

medical care provision by a physician of services related to the maintenance of health, prevention of illness, and treatment of illness or injury

medical care institution institution with permanent facilities and an organized professional staff that provides medical services to patients

medical care unit See *inpatient care unit*

medical center hospital usually affiliated with a medical school, or group of hospitals located within a limited geographic area and usually affiliated with a medical school, that provides a broad range of medical and health-related services to patients

medical computer specialist person who develops data processing systems and programs for analysis and interpretation of medical and related data

medical consultation upon request by one physician, another physician's review of a patient's history, examination of the patient, and recommendations

medical director physician, usually employed by a hospital, who serves in a medical and administrative capacity as head of the organized medical staff and who also may serve as liaison for the medical staff with the administration and governing board See also *chief of staff*

medical education, director of member of the medical staff of a hospital or an educator who coordinates its programs of graduate and continuing medical education

medical engineering field of study that uses biomedical engineering and technological concepts to develop equipment and instruments required in health care delivery

medical illustrator artist qualified by special training in medical illustration who illustrates medical phenomena

medical indigence See *indigence, medical*

medical laboratory assistant See *medical laboratory technician, medical technologist*

medical laboratory technician person who, under the supervision of a medical technologist, pathologist, or physician, performs chemical, microscopic, and bacteriological tests of human blood, tissue, and fluids for diagnostic and research purposes

medical photographer photographer qualified by special training in the biological sciences who photographs medical phenomena

medical record record of a patient maintained by a hospital or a physician for the purpose of documenting clinical data on diagnosis, treatment, and outcome

medical record, problem-oriented methodology for accumulating, organizing, and delineating patient data by each of the problems presented See also *medical record*

medical record administrator person who maintains records that meet the medical, administrative, legal, ethical, regulatory, and institutional requirements of a hospital See also *registered record administrator*

medical record analyst person who, under the supervision of a medical record administrator or medical staff committee, abstracts and compiles data from patients' medical records

medical record department department providing systems and services for filing, maintenance, security, and retrieval of primary and secondary medical records; for collecting, coding, and indexing health care data; for processing authorized disclosure of medical record information; for quantitative analysis of medical records; and for preparation of administrative and clinical statistical reports

medical record librarian See *medical record administrator*

medical record technician person who, under the supervision of a medical record administrator, provides technical skills necessary to maintain records that meet the medical, administrative, ethical, legal, accreditation, and regulatory requirements of a hospital

medical secretary person who prepares and maintains departmental medical records and performs related secretarial duties

medical services activities related to medical care performed by physicians, nurses, and other professional and technical personnel under the direction of a physician

medical staff aggregate body of licensed medical and osteopathic physicians and dentists who have been accorded the privilege of caring for patients of a hospital

medical staff, active physicians and dentists on the medical staff who regularly provide medical practice within the hospital and who participate in all medical staff activities

medical staff, associate physicians and dentists who have applied for appointment to the medical staff and who, for an interim period, are accorded the privilege of admitting patients but whose participation in medical staff activities is limited in accordance with medical staff bylaws

medical staff, courtesy physicians and dentists who meet qualifications for appointment to the medical staff but who admit patients to the hospital only occasionally or act only as consultants and who are ineligible to participate in medical staff activities

medical staff, honorary physicians and dentists, usually retired, who are recognized by the medical staff for their noteworthy contributions but who may not admit patients to the hospital or participate in medical staff activities

medical staff, organized formal organization of the medical staff of a hospital that has been delegated responsibility and authority to maintain proper standards of medical care within the institution

medical student person who is enrolled in a program of study to fulfill requirements for a doctorate of medicine

medical technologist person who, under the direction of a pathologist, other physician, or scientist, performs specialized chemical, microscopic, and bacteriological tests of human blood, tissue, and fluids

medical technologist, certified medical technologist who has successfully completed the examination of the Board of Registry of the American Society of Clinical Pathologists, the American Medical Technologists, the International Society of Clinical Laboratory Technologists, the National Certification Agency for Medical Laboratory Personnel, or the Proficiency Examination of the Department of Health and Human Services See also *medical technologist*

medical transcriptionist person who transcribes reports for patients' medical records

Medicare federal program, created by Title XVIII—Health Insurance for the Aged, a 1965 amendment to the Social Security Act, that provides health insurance benefits primarily to persons over the age of 65 and others eligible for Social Security benefits

medication order written order by a physician or a dentist or other designated professional for medication to be dispensed by a hospital pharmacy for administration to an inpatient See also *prescription*

merger formal combination of two or more hospitals into a single new legal entity that has the identity of one of the preexisting hospitals See also *consolidation*

microbiologist, medical microbiologist or bacteriologist who identifies microorganisms found in patients

microbiology laboratory laboratory for examination of tissue and other specimens by means of microbiologic tests

microbiology technologist medical technologist who specializes in identification of bacteria and other microorganisms See also *medical technologist*

midwife See *nurse, midwife*

minimal care unit unit for the treatment of inpatients who are ambulatory and able to meet many of their own daily living needs and require only minimal nursing care

morgue unit providing for storage and autopsy of dead persons

mortality rate See *death rate*

multihospital system two or more hospitals, owned, leased, sponsored, or contract-managed by a central organization

multi-institutional arrangement two or more institutions organized in a particular way or for a specific purpose

multiphasic screening systematic gathering of patient health data and administration of comprehensive clinical examinations, usually by paramedical personnel and utilizing automated instrumentation, for the purpose of detecting early stages of illness

municipal hospital See *hospital, municipal*

music therapist person who uses music as a therapeutic agent for patients

Nn

national health insurance federal health insurance program to provide comprehensive benefits to the majority of the population

neighborhood health center See *community health center*

neonatal intensive care unit See *intensive care unit, neonatal*

neonatal unit See *nursery, newborn*

neurologist physician who specializes in the diagnosis and treatment of diseases of the nervous system

neurosurgeon surgeon who specializes in the surgical treatment of diseases of the nervous system

newborn intensive care unit See *intensive care unit, neonatal*

night bed See *bed, night*

night care program organizational entity that provides services to patients who, for therapeutic purposes, use hospital facilities on a regularly scheduled basis for a substantial number of nighttime hours but do not require inpatient care 24 hours a day

night hospital See *hospital, night*

nonfederal government hospital See *hospital, nonfederal government*

nonmaternal death See *death, nonmaternal*

nosocomial originating in a hospital, used with reference to infection

nosocomial infection See *infection, nosocomial*

not-for-profit hospital See *hospital, not-for-profit*

nuclear medicine physician physician who specializes in the diagnosis and treatment of disease through the use of radioisotopes

nuclear medicine service service providing diagnosis and treatment through use of radioisotopes

nuclear medicine technician person who assists physicians in the detection of disease through the use of scanning devices using radioisotopes See also *medical laboratory technician*

nurse person qualified by a formal nursing program at an accredited school of nursing who, under the supervision of a physician, provides nursing services to patients requiring assistance in recovering or maintaining their physical or mental health See also *nurse, registered*

nurse, cardiac care staff nurse qualified by advanced training in cardiac care who provides care to cardiac patients

25

nurse, charge registered nurse who directs and supervises the provision of nursing care in one patient care unit for the duration of one shift See also *nurse, head*

nurse, circulating registered nurse qualified by specialized training in operating room techniques who is responsible for establishing and maintaining a safe, therapeutic environment for patients during surgery

nurse, critical care registered nurse qualified by advanced training in critical care who provides care to critically ill patients

nurse, float nurse who is assigned to duty on an as-needed basis, usually to assist in times of unusually heavy work loads or to assume the duties of absent nursing personnel See also *float pool*

nurse, general-duty See *nurse, staff*

nurse, head registered nurse who, as an ongoing responsibility, directs and manages the nursing care activities of one patient care unit See also *nurse, charge*

nurse, infection control registered nurse who performs surveillance and infection prevention and control activities

nurse, licensed practical person qualified by an approved program in practical or vocational nursing and licensed by the state who, under the direction of a head nurse or nursing team leader, performs a variety of assigned nursing activities

nurse, licensed vocational See *nurse, licensed practical*

nurse, operating room registered nurse qualified by postgraduate or on-the-job training who assists surgeons and anesthesiologists in the performance of surgical procedures

nurse, primary registered nurse who provides all nursing care to assigned patients throughout their hospitalization

nurse, private-duty registered nurse who, as an independent contractor employed by the patient, provides direct nursing care to the patient

nurse, psychiatric registered nurse qualified by specialized training who provides nursing care to patients with mental illness

nurse, registered person qualified by an approved postsecondary program or baccalaureate in nursing and licensed by the state to practice nursing

nurse, scrub registered nurse or operating room technician who assists surgeons during surgery

nurse, staff registered nurse who is responsible for assessing, planning, implementing, and evaluating the care of designated patients

nurse, student person enrolled in a nursing education program

nurse, team registered nurse or licensed practical nurse who is a member of a nursing team See also *team nursing*

nurse anesthetist registered nurse, usually qualified by an accredited educational program in anesthesiology, who, under the supervision of a physician or dentist, administers anesthetic agents to patients before and during surgery and assists in management and resuscitation of critical patients in intensive care, coronary care, and emergency situations

nurse anesthetist, certified registered nurse anesthetist certified by the Council on Certification/Council on Recertification of Nurse Anesthetists as meeting the stated requirements for certification/recertification

nurse anesthetist, licensed See *nurse anesthetist*

nurse anesthetist, qualified See *nurse anesthetist*

nurse clinical instructor registered nurse who teaches and supervises nursing students in a clinical area

nurse clinician registered nurse qualified by advanced training in a nursing specialty who practices, teaches, consults, supervises, or coordinates nursing services in that specialty See also *nurse specialist, clinical*

nurse coordinator registered nurse who coordinates and manages the activities of nursing personnel engaged in specific nursing services, such as obstetrics or surgery, for two or more patient care units See also *patient care coordinator, utilization review coordinator*

nurse epidemiologist See *epidemiologist, nurse*

nurse midwife registered nurse qualified by advanced training in obstetric and neonatal care and certified by the American College of Nurse Midwives who manages the perinatal care of women having normal pregnancy, labor, and childbirth

nurse practitioner registered nurse qualified by a baccalaureate or formal educational preparation who, under the supervision of a physician, engages in health care evaluation and decision making related to patient care

nurse specialist, clinical registered nurse qualified by a graduate degree in a nursing specialty who practices, teaches, consults in, supervises, or coordinates nursing care in that specialty See also *nurse clinician*

nurse supervisor See *patient care coordinator*

nurse therapist See *nurse, primary*

nursery See *nursery, newborn*

nursery, newborn unit for care and treatment of newborn infants through the age of 28 days or longer if necessary

nursery, premature unit for care and treatment of infants who were born prematurely or whose birth weight is 2,500 grams or less

nursing See *nursing care*

nursing administrator See *nursing service administrator*

nursing aide See *nursing assistant*

nursing assistant person who, under the supervision of a registered nurse, performs routine personal care activities

nursing attendant See *nursing assistant*

nursing care provision of services by or under the direction of a nurse to patients requiring assistance in recovering or maintaining their physical or mental health

nursing care facility See *nursing home*

nursing care institution See *nursing home*

nursing care plan formal, written plan of the nursing care activities to be conducted on behalf of a given patient and used to coordinate the activities of all nursing personnel involved in that patient's care

nursing care unit See *inpatient care unit*

nursing differential allowance added to payments to hospitals for services rendered Medicare patients in recognition of the greater cost of providing nursing services to these patients than to the general patient population

nursing director See *nursing service administrator*

nursing home institution with an organized professional staff and permanent facilities, including inpatient beds, that provides continuous nursing and other health-related, psychosocial, and personal services to patients who are not in an acute phase of illness but who primarily require continued care on an inpatient basis

nursing home administrator person licensed by the state who is responsible for the management or administration of a nursing home

nursing service service providing nursing care to patients

nursing service administrator registered nurse responsible for the overall administration and management of nursing services provided in a hospital

nursing service director See *nursing service administrator*

nursing services activities related to nursing care performed by nurses and other professional and technical personnel under the supervision of a registered nurse

nursing team group of registered nurses and auxiliary nursing personnel who implement total nursing care programs planned by the team leader for designated patients

nursing team leader registered nurse who directs the patient care activities of a nursing team

nutritionist See *dietitian, clinical*

nutritionist, clinical See *dietitian, clinical*

Oo

obstetrician physician who specializes in the care and medical and surgical treatment of pregnant women

occasion of service specific identifiable act of service provided a patient, such as performance of a test, medical examination, treatment, or procedure

occupancy ratio of average daily census to the average number of beds maintained during the reporting period

occupational therapist person qualified by an approved program and licensed by the state who plans and implements programs to restore, develop, or maintain the task performance skills necessary to permit patients to perform daily living tasks

occupational therapy treatment, by means of constructive activities, to restore, develop, or maintain the skills necessary to permit physically and mentally disabled persons to perform daily living tasks

occupational therapy aide person who, under the supervision of an occupational therapist, performs clerical and related tasks necessary for the implementation of occupational therapy programs

occupational therapy assistant person who, under the supervision of an occupational therapist, assists in the implementation of occupational therapy

occupational therapy department service providing assistance to patients in restoring, developing, or maintaining skills necessary to permit them to perform daily living tasks

occupied bed day See *day, occupied bed*

ombudsman See *patient representative*

oncologist physician who specializes in the diagnosis and treatment of cancer

oncology service service providing treatment to patients with cancer

one-to-one care method of organizing nursing services in an inpatient care unit by which one registered nurse assumes responsibility for all nursing care provided one patient for the duration of one shift

operating room unit for the performance of surgery

operating room nurse See *nurse, operating room*

operating room technician person who performs certain functions related to ensuring the cleanliness, safety, and efficiency of the operating room See also *nurse, scrub*

operating room technician, certified operating room technician certified by the Association of Operating Room Technicians

ophthalmologist physician who specializes in the diagnosis and treatment of diseases and defects of the eye and related structures

organized professional staff formal organization of the professional personnel of a hospital that includes one or more physicians and to which is delegated the authority and responsibility for maintaining proper standards of medical care and/or health-related care

orthoptist person qualified by a postsecondary training program and examination by the American Orthoptist Council who, under the supervision of an ophthalmologist, tests eye muscles and teaches exercises designed to correct eye coordination defects

orthotics assistant person who, under the supervision of an orthotist, assists in the design and fitting of braces and other orthopedic appliances

orthotics technician person who assists an orthotist in the fabrication of braces and other orthopedic appliances

orthotist person who designs, fabricates, and fits braces and other orthopedic appliances prescribed by physicians

orthotist, certified orthotist who has successfully completed the examination of the American Orthotist and Prosthetic Association See also *orthotist*

osteopath physician who specializes in a system of medical practice based on the theory that disease is due chiefly to loss of structural integrity, which can be restored by manipulation of the parts of the body and supplemented by therapeutic measures, such as medicine and surgery

OT See *occupational therapy, occupational therapist*

otolaryngologist physician who specializes in the diagnosis and treatment of diseases and injuries of the ears, nose, and throat

outpatient person who receives medical, dental, or other health-related services in a hospital or other health care institution but who is not lodged there

outpatient, general clinic See *outpatient service*

outpatient, specialty clinic See *outpatient service*

outpatient care See *ambulatory care*

outpatient clinic See *outpatient service*

outpatient department See *outpatient service*

outpatient service service providing treatment to patients who do not require admission as inpatients

outpatient visit all services provided an outpatient in the course of a single appearance in an outpatient or inpatient unit

Pp

PA See *physician's assistant*

paramedic See *emergency medical technician-paramedic*

paramedical personnel nonphysicians who work in the health field, including but not limited to medical technicians, aides, nutritionists, and physician's assistants

partial hospitalization program organizational entity that provides therapeutic services to patients who use day or night hospital facilities or adult day health services on a regularly scheduled basis

pastoral counseling department See *chaplaincy service*

pathologist physician who specializes in the study of the origin and course of disease and whose practice is conducted chiefly in the laboratory, performing postmortem and research studies

pathologist, anatomic pathologist who specializes in the gross and microscopic study of organs and tissues removed for biopsy or during postmortem examinations See also *pathologist*

pathologist, clinical pathologist who specializes in the study of disease-induced and physiological changes in body fluids and tissues as they pertain to treatment of disease See also *pathologist*

pathology laboratory See *pathology service*

pathology service service providing for the study and diagnosis of disease through laboratory examination of body tissues and fluids

patient person who receives a health care service from a provider

patient, bed patient who is not ambulatory

patient, emergency patient with potentially disabling or life-threatening condition who receives initial evaluation and medical, dental, or other health-related service in an emergency department

patient accounts manager person who directs the activities of personnel engaged in credit and collection functions

patient advocate See *patient representative*

patient care audit See *audit, patient care*

patient care committee hospital committee composed of medical, nursing, and other professional staff members whose purpose is to monitor all patient care practices and ensure that predetermined standards are met

patient care coordinator registered nurse who manages and directs a specific nursing service, such as obstetrics, pediatrics, or surgery, for two or more patient care units See also *nurse coordinator*

patient care plan See *care plan, nursing care plan*

patient care unit See *inpatient care unit*

patient compensation fund fund established by state law and most commonly financed by placing a surcharge on malpractice premiums of all professional liability policyholders in the state and used to pay malpractice claims

patient education department department providing patients and their families with instruction related to health maintenance and the management of illness and disability See also *education department*

patient representative person who investigates and mediates patients' problems and complaints in relation to a hospital's services

patient representative services services provided by designated staff related to the investigation and mediation of patients' problems and complaints and to the promotion and protection of patients' rights

pediatrician physician who specializes in the care and treatment of children from birth to adolescence

pediatrics service service providing diagnosis and treatment of patients usually under the age of 14

peer review See *review, peer*

peer review committee committee composed of practicing physicians appointed or elected by a medical society whose purpose is to evaluate the quality and efficiency of patient care practices of physicians

per diem rate See *rate, per diem*

perfusion technologist person who, under the supervision of a physician, operates a heart-lung machine used for cardiopulmonary bypass during surgery

permanent fund See *fund, endowment*

personal care institution See *residential care facility*

personal care services services performed to assist patients in meeting the requirements of daily living

pharmacist person qualified by a baccalaureate or graduate degree in pharmacy and licensed by the state who prepares, dispenses, and provides for the control of prescription drugs

pharmacologist person qualified by a graduate degree in pharmacology who conducts research to develop drugs

pharmacy department department controlling the preparation, dispensing, storage, and use of drugs

pharmacy technician person who assists a pharmacist in technical, nonjudgmental duties, such as compounding and packaging drugs

philanthropy director See *development, director of*

phlebotomist person, usually a nurse or medical laboratory technologist, who draws blood from patients and blood donors

physiatrist physician who specializes in evaluation of the rehabilitation needs and management of the rehabilitation programs of disabled persons

physical medicine use of physical therapy techniques to return physically diseased or injured patients to a useful life

physical medicine service service providing physical therapy and other physical restorative and maintenance programs See also *rehabilitation service*

physical therapist person qualified by an approved certificate program or baccalaureate in physical therapy and licensed by the state who treats disease and injury by physical means, such as the application of light, heat, cold, water, electricity, massage, and exercise

physical therapy treatment of disease and injury by physical means such as massage, exercise, heat, cold, water, and electricity

physical therapy aide person who, under the supervision of a physical therapist, assists in carrying out patient treatment programs and performing related clerical tasks

physical therapy assistant person who, under the supervision of a physical therapist, assists in carrying out patient treatment programs and performs related maintenance and clerical tasks

physical therapy department service providing for treatment of disease and injury by physical means such as massage, exercise, heat, cold, water, electricity, light, and ultrasound

physician person qualified by a doctorate in medicine or osteopathy and licensed by the state to practice medicine

physician, attending member of a hospital medical staff who is legally responsible for the care provided a given patient

physician, contract member of a hospital medical staff or other physician who, under a full-time or part-time contract, provides care in the hospital and whose payment as defined in the contract may be an institutional responsibility, on a fee basis, or on another agreed-on basis

physician, critical care physician who cares for the critically ill and injured at the scene of an emergency or during transport to a hospital and who in the hospital provides prolonged intensive medical and surgical care

physician, emergency department physician who specializes in the immediate initial evaluation, care, and disposition of patients with acute illness or injury and who works in a hospital emergency department on a salaried or a contract basis

physician, full-time See *physician, hospital-based*

physician, geographic full-time physician whose primary source of income is a salary received for services to a hospital and who also engages in clinical practice at that hospital See also *physician, salaried*

physician, hospital-based physician, such as a director of medical education, pathologist, radiologist, or emergency department physician, who spends a predominant part of his or her practice time within one or more hospitals

physician, primary care physician who specializes in general internal medicine, general pediatrics, family practice, or obstetrics/gynecology

physician, resident graduate of an accredited medical school participating in an approved training program in a hospital setting

physician, salaried physician who is employed by a hospital on a salaried basis

physician extender physician's assistant, nurse practitioner, or other health care professional trained in a paramedical discipline who, under the supervision of a physician, performs patient care services See also *physician's assistant, nurse practitioner*

physician's assistant person who assists a physician by performing delegated tasks, such as taking medical histories and performing physical examinations

physician's associate See *physician's assistant*

plan of care See *care plan*

planning agency See *health systems agency; state health planning and development agency*

plant engineer See *engineer, chief*

podiatric service service providing diagnosis and treatment to patients with foot disorders or injuries or anatomic defects of the foot

podiatrist person qualified by an accredited program in podiatric medicine and licensed by the state who diagnoses and treats foot diseases and deformities by medical, surgical, and physical means

policy adjustment See *administrative adjustment*

postoperative care provision of medical, nursing, and other health-related services to patients following surgery

postoperative recovery room See *recovery room*

postpartum care provision of medical, nursing, and other health-related services to patients following childbirth

postsurgical care See *postoperative care*

preadmission process for admission See *admission, preadmission process for*

preoperative care physiological and psychological preparation of a patient for surgery

prepayment payment in advance by subscribers to a third party (e.g., Blue Cross) for health care services that may be provided in the future and that will be paid for by the third party after the services have been provided

prescription, drug written order by a physician, dentist, or other designated professional for medication to be dispensed by a pharmacy for use by a patient See also *medication order*

president See *chief executive officer*

president of medical staff member of a hospital medical staff who is elected or appointed by the medical staff to serve as its administrative head for a designated time See also *chief of staff*

primary care provision by a primary care physician of those medical services required to maintain the health of a well person or restore the health of a patient suffering from an illness See also *physician, primary care; secondary care; tertiary care*

primary care physician See *physician, primary care*

primary nurse See *nurse, primary*

primary nursing method of organizing nursing services within a hospital inpatient care unit by which one registered nurse assumes responsibility for all nursing care provided a group of designated patients throughout the duration of their hospitalization

prison hospital See *hospital, security*

private hospital See *hospital, private*

private room hospital room designed and equipped to house one inpatient

private-duty nurse See *nurse, private-duty*

privileges, clinical formal authority granted to a physician or a dentist by a hospital governing board to provide care to patients within limits based on the physician's or dentist's professional license, experience, and competence

privileges, emergency temporary authority granted to a physician or a dentist by a hospital governing board or chief executive officer to provide care to patients in an emergency situation within limits based on the physician's or dentist's professional license and without regard to regular service assignment or staff status

privileges, temporary temporary authority granted to a physician or a dentist by a hospital governing board to provide care to patients for a limited period or to a specific patient for that patient's hospitalization within limits based on the physician's or dentist's professional license, experience, and competence

product evaluation committee hospital committee composed of medical, nursing, purchasing, and administrative staff members whose purpose is to evaluate products and advise on their procurement

professional liability obligation of a health care professional or a hospital to use due care in the conduct of a professional service, for a breach of which the law provides a remedy

professional liability insurance insurance that protects providers against loss incurred as the result of judgments for damages resulting from findings of failure of a health care professional to use due care in the conduct of a professional service

professional standards review organization physician-sponsored organization with designated authority to review the medical necessity, appropriateness, and quality of services provided under the Medicare, Medicaid, and Maternal and Child Health programs

progressive patient care method of organizing nursing services within a hospital by which patients are grouped into levels of inpatient care units—usually, intensive, intermediate, and self-care units—according to their degree of illness

proprietary hospital See *hospital, investor-owned*

prosector person who, under the supervision of a pathologist, performs gross dissections and prepares autopsy specimens for pathological examination

prospective reimbursement See *reimbursement, prospective*

prospective review See *review, prospective*

prosthetics assistant person who, under the supervision of a prosthetist, assists in the design and fitting of artificial limbs

prosthetics technician person who assists a prosthetist in the fabrication of artificial limbs

prosthetist person who fabricates and fits artificial limbs prescribed by physicians

prosthetist, certified prosthetist who has successfully completed the examination of the American Orthotic and Prosthetic Association See also *prosthetist*

provider hospital or health care professional or group of hospitals or health care professionals that provide health care services to patients

PSRO See *professional standards review organization*

psychiatric aide See *psychiatric technician*

psychiatric care provision by or under the direction of a psychiatrist of services related to the diagnosis and treatment of mental illness

psychiatric emergency service service providing immediate initial evaluation and treatment to acutely mentally or emotionally disturbed patients available on a 24-hour-a-day basis

psychiatric foster care observation and care of a patient in an approved foster home usually following discharge as a psychiatric inpatient

psychiatric home care observation and care of a patient in his or her place of residence, which may follow discharge as a psychiatric inpatient

psychiatric hospital See *hospital, psychiatric*

psychiatric inpatient unit unit for treatment of inpatients who require psychiatric care

psychiatric nurse See *nurse, psychiatric*

psychiatric services provision of psychiatric care performed by physicians, nurses, and other professional and trained technical personnel under the direction of a psychiatrist

psychiatric technician person who, under the supervision of a psychiatrist, psychologist, social worker, or nurse, assists in carrying out prescribed treatment plans for emotionally ill patients

psychiatrist physician who specializes in the study, diagnosis, and treatment of mental, emotional, and behavioral disorders

psychologist, clinical person qualified by a graduate degree in psychology and training in clinical psychology who studies the behavior of individuals and groups and who provides testing and counseling services to patients with mental and emotional disorders

psychotherapist psychiatrist, clinical psychologist, psychiatric social worker, or other person professionally trained to practice psychotherapy See *psychiatrist; psychologist, clinical; social worker, psychiatric*

psychotherapy treatment of mental, emotional, and behavioral disorders by means of verbal or nonverbal communication with the patient

PT See *physical therapy, physical therapist*

public affairs, director of See *public relations, director of*

public affairs department See *public relations department*

public information department See *public relations department*

public information officer See *public relations, director of*

public relations, director of person who plans and implements programs to communicate with the hospital's audiences and to enhance the public's perception of the hospital

public relations department department responsible for news media relations, special events, reports, publications, and promotional materials

pulmonary function laboratory laboratory for examination and evaluation of patients' respiratory functions by means of electromechanical equipment

purchasing, director of person who is responsible for the procurement of supplies and equipment See also *materials manager*

purchasing agent See *purchasing, director of*

purchasing department department providing for purchasing of equipment and supplies See also *materials management department*

Qq

QAP See *quality assurance program*

qualified formally recognized by an appropriate agency or organization as meeting certain standards of performance related to the professional competence of an individual or the eligibility of an institution to participate in a government program

quality assurance program review of selected hospital medical records by medical staff members, performed for the purposes of evaluating the quality and effectiveness of medical care in relation to accepted standards and of planning continuing education activities for the medical staff

Rr

radiation therapist See *health physicist*

radioisotope facility See *nuclear medicine service*

radiation therapy treatment of disease by means of X rays or other forms of radiant energy

radiologic technologist person who, usually under the supervision of a radiologist, operates radiologic equipment and assists radiologists and other physicians

radiologic technologist, certified radiologic technologist certified by the Joint Review Committee on Education and Radiologic Technology of the American College of Radiology and the American Society of Radiologic Technologists

radiologist physician who specializes in the diagnosis and treatment of disease by means of X rays and other forms of radiant energy

radiology service service providing diagnosis and treatment through the use of X rays and other forms of radiant energy

radium therapy treatment of disease through the use of radium

rate, inclusive prospectively established rate of payment that assigns a single charge to a day of inpatient care regardless of the number or intensity of services provided

rate, interim amount periodically paid to a provider by a third-party payer under a retrospective reimbursement arrangement

rate, per diem established rate of payment determined by dividing the total cost of providing routine inpatient services for a given period by the total number of inpatient days of care provided during that period

rate review See *review, rate*

rate setting process of establishing rates for hospital services by taking into account the financial needs of the hospital See also *review, rate*

RD registered dietitian See *dietitian, registered*

recovery room room for monitoring and treating postoperative patients

recreational therapist See *therapeutic recreation specialist*

registered hospital See *hospital, registered*

registered nurse See *nurse, registered*

registered record administrator medical record administrator who has successfully completed the credentialing examination conducted by the American Medical Record Association See also *medical record administrator*

rehabilitation center See *rehabilitation facility*

rehabilitation counselor person who counsels disabled persons in attaining their maximum functional capacity

rehabilitation facility facility that provides medical, health-related, social, and/or vocational services to disabled persons to help them attain their maximum functional capacity

rehabilitation hospital See *rehabilitation facility*

rehabilitation program organizational entity that provides medical, health-related, social, and/or vocational services to disabled persons to help them attain their maximum functional capacity

rehabilitation service service providing medical, health-related, social and/or vocational services to help disabled persons attain and/or retain their maximum functional capacity

rehabilitation unit unit for treatment of inpatients who require assistance in attaining and/or retaining their maximum functional capacity

rehabilitative care provision, under the supervision of a physician, of coordinated medical, health-related, social, and/or vocational services to physically, mentally, or emotionally disabled persons

rehabilitative services medical, health-related, social, and/or vocational services performed by professional and technical personnel to help physically, mentally, or emotionally disabled persons attain and/or retain their functional capacity

reimbursement, cost-based payment by a third-party payer to a hospital of all allowable costs incurred by the hospital in the provision of services to patients covered by the contract

reimbursement, prospective method of third-party payment by which costs to be incurred by an institution in providing services to patients are based not on actual costs but on estimates made at the beginning of a fiscal period See also *reimbursement, retrospective*

reimbursement, retroactive additional payment by a third-party payer to an institution for services not identified at the time of initial reimbursement See also *reimbursement, retrospective*

reimbursement, retrospective method of third-party payment by which costs incurred by a hospital in providing services to covered patients are based on actual costs determined at the end of a fiscal period See also *reimbursement, prospective*; *reimbursement, retroactive*

reimbursement specialist person who prepares materials to obtain third-party reimbursement and who may negotiate reimbursement structures with third-party payers

relative value unit unit of measure designed to permit comparison of the amounts of resources required to perform various services within a single department or between similar departments in various hospitals by assigning weight to such factors as personnel time, level of skill, and sophistication of equipment required to render service

renal dialysis unit See *hemodialysis unit*

resident, administrative student in an accredited program in hospital or health care administration who participates in a practical training experience in a health care institution

resident, long-term person who is not in an acute phase of illness but who requires primarily convalescent, restorative, or continuing nursing care

resident, medical specialty physician in training who participates in an accredited program of graduate medical education sponsored by a hospital

resident physician See *physician, resident*

residential care facility facility that provides custodial care to persons who, because of their physical, mental, or emotional condition, are not able to live independently

respiratory diseases unit unit for treatment of inpatients with respiratory diseases

respiratory therapist person who, under the supervision of a physician, administers oxygen and other gases and provides assistance to patients with breathing difficulties

respiratory therapist, registered respiratory therapist who has successfully completed the examination of the National Board of Respiratory Therapy See also *respiratory therapist*

respiratory therapy treatment of breathing disorders through administration of oxygen and other gases and teaching of breathing exercises

respiratory therapy aide See *respiratory therapy assistant*

respiratory therapy assistant person who assists a respiratory therapist through such activities as maintaining equipment and transporting patients

respiratory therapy service service providing for treatment of patients with breathing disorders

respiratory therapy technician person who, under the supervision of a physician, treats patients with cardiorespiratory problems through the administration of oxygen and other gases

respiratory therapy technician, certified respiratory therapy technician who has successfully completed the examination of the National Board for Respiratory Therapy See also *respiratory therapy technician*

restricted funds See *funds, restricted*

retirement center facility or organized program that provides social services and activities to retired persons who generally do not require ongoing health care

retroactive reimbursement See *reimbursement, retroactive*

retrospective reimbursement See *reimbursement, retrospective*

retrospective review See *audit, medical*

review, admissions review of the medical necessity of a patient's admission to a hospital, conducted at or shortly after admission

review, capital expenditure prospective review by a designated state regulatory agency of the appropriateness of capital expenditures proposed by hospitals in a designated area

review, claims retrospective review by a third-party payer of a request for payment, performed for the purpose of determining the liability of the payer, eligibility of the beneficiary and the provider, and appropriateness of the service provided and amount requested under an insurance or prepayment contract

review, concurrent evaluation of the medical necessity of a patient's admission to a hospital, conducted at or shortly after admission, and the periodic evaluation thereafter of the appropriateness of services provided during the patient's hospitalization, performed for the purpose of determining appropriate payment for services

review, continued-stay review of the appropriateness of the continued hospitalization of a patient

review, peer concurrent of retrospective review by practicing physicians or other health professionals of the quality and efficiency of patient care practices or services ordered or performed by other physicians or other health professionals

review, prospective evaluation of the medical necessity of a patient's admission to a hospital conducted prior to the admission

review, rate prospective review by a government or private agency of a hospital's budget and financial data, performed for the purpose of determining the reasonableness of the hospital rates and evaluating proposed rate increases

review, retrospective See *audit, medical*

review, utilization concurrent or retrospective review of the appropriateness of admissions, medical and supportive services rendered, and lengths of stay

risk management function of planning, organizing, and directing a comprehensive program of activities to identify, evaluate, and take corrective action against risks that may lead to patient injury, employee injury, and property loss or damage with resulting financial loss

risk manager person who coordinates all aspects of risk identification, evaluation, and treatment within the hospital in order to reduce the frequency and severity of events that may result in injury to patients, visitors, and employees and in property loss or damage

RN See *nurse, registered*

room rate See *charge, daily service*

rooming-in method of organizing obstetric facilities and services whereby mothers share accommodations with and assume the care of newborn infants under the supervision of nursing personnel

RRA See *registered record administrator*

Ss

safety committee committee composed of medical, nursing, engineering, administrative, and other staff members whose purpose is to oversee safety practices

safety director qualified person who oversees those activities related to ensuring a hospital's functional safety, such as its fire prevention, environmental safety, and disaster planning activities

satellite hospital See *hospital, satellite*

scrub nurse See *nurse, scrub*

second opinion examination and evaluation by a surgeon of a patient recommended for surgery by another surgeon

second-opinion program elective or mandatory medical review mechanism established by a health benefit program to encourage the provision of second opinions See also *second opinion*

secondary care provision of a specialized medical service by a physician specialist or a hospital, usually upon referral by a primary care physician

Section 1122 section of the Social Security Act added by the Social Security Amendments of 1972 (Public Law 93-603) that denies payment under Medicare and Medicaid for certain capital expenditures not approved by state planning agencies

security department department providing for the security and safety of patients, employees, medical staff, visitors, and their property while in the hospital or on its grounds

security director person who is responsible for a program to protect a hospital against fire, theft, violence, illegal entry, and other hazards to the security and safety of people and property

security guard person who guards entrances and corridors to protect a hospital against fire, theft, violence, illegal entry, and other hazards to the security and safety of people and property

security hospital See *hospital, security*

self-care unit See *minimal care unit*

self-insurance means by which hospitals or professionals may, in lieu of commercial insurance, assume financial responsibility for liability

semiprivate room room designed and equipped to house two to four inpatients

serologist bacteriologist who prepares or supervises the preparation of serums used to diagnose and treat diseases and to immunize persons against diseases

serology technologist medical technologist who prepares serums used to diagnose and treat diseases and immunize persons against disease See also *medical technologist*

services, routine room, board, and medical and nursing services regularly provided to patients in the course of care

shared services administrative, clinical, or service functions that are common to two or more health care institutions, which are used jointly or cooperatively by them in some manner for the purpose of improving service, containing cost, and/or effecting economies of scale

shared services organization separate legal entity established by two or more organizations or institutions that allows joint control by sponsoring organizations or institutions

SHCC See *statewide health coordinating council*

sheltered care home See *residential care facility*

sheltered care institution See *residential care facility*

shared care services provision of personal care, supervision, an activities program, and in some instances medical care to persons who require assistance in meeting their daily living needs but do not require continuing nursing care

sheltered workshop facility or program, either for outpatients or for residents within an institutional setting, that provides work experience in a controlled working environment and related vocational rehabilitation services to persons with physical or mental disabilities

short-term hospital See *hospital, short-term*

SHPDA See *state health planning and development agency*

skilled nursing care nursing and/or other rehabilitation services provided to Medicare beneficiaries by or under the supervision of professional or technical personnel under conditions prescribed by the Medicare program

skilled nursing facility facility with an organized professional staff that, under a transfer agreement with one or more hospitals, provides medical, continuous nursing, and various other health and social services to patients who are not in an acute phase of illness but who require primarily restorative or skilled nursing care on an inpatient basis

skilled nursing unit unit that provides physician services and continuous professional nursing supervision for patients who are not in an acute phase of illness but who require primarily restorative or skilled nursing care

social services See *social work*

social work assistance to patients and their families in dealing with social, emotional, and environmental problems associated with illness or disability, performed by or under the supervision of a social worker

social work aide See *social work assistant*

social work assistant person who, under the supervision of a social worker, assists individuals and their families in dealing with psychosocial and/or environmental problems resulting from illness or disability

social work service service providing assistance and counseling to patients and their families in dealing with social, emotional, and environmental problems

social worker, hospital social worker who, working in a hospital, counsels and assists individuals and their families in dealing with social, emotional, and/or environmental problems resulting from illness or disability

social worker, medical social worker qualified by a master's degree who, working in a health care setting, counsels and assists individuals and their families in dealing with social, emotional, and/or environmental problems resulting from illness or disability

social worker, psychiatric social worker qualified by a master's degree who, working in a psychiatric hospital or psychiatric unit of a general hospital or mental health center, counsels and assists individuals and their families in dealing with social, emotional, and/or environmental problems resulting from mental illness or disability

special care unit unit, such as burn care unit, intensive care unit, or cardiac care unit, for treatment of critically ill patients

specialty hospital See *hospital, specialty*

specialist physician, dentist, or other health professional, usually with special advanced education and training, who limits his or her practice to specific services, procedures, diseases, or categories of patients

specialty care provision by a physician specialist of specialized medical services

specific-purpose fund See *fund, specific-purpose*

speech pathologist person who treats speech and language disorders

speech pathology service service providing evaluation and treatment to patients with speech and language disorders

spell of illness under Medicare, that period that elapses between the day on which the insured patient enters a hospital and the day that marks the end of a 60-consecutive-day period during which the insured has not been an inpatient of a hospital or skilled nursing facility

staff development See *education, in-service*

staff nurse See *nurse, staff*

staff privileges See *privileges, clinical*

state health planning and development agency unit of state government organized in accordance with the Health Planning and Resources Development Act of 1974 (Public Law 93-641) to perform various health planning and development functions, including administration of the state's certificate-of-need programs and preparation of a statewide health plan See also *statewide health coordinating council, health systems agency*

statewide health coordinating council organization of health care providers and consumers designated by a state in accordance with the Health Planning and Resources Development Act of 1974 (Public Law 93-641) to coordinate the activities of the state health planning and development agency and the health systems agencies in the state, including approval of the statewide health plan See also *state health planning and development agency, health systems agency*

student nurse See *nurse, student*

superintendent See *chief executive officer*

supervisory nurse See *patient care coordinator*

surgeon physician who specializes in the surgical treatment of diseases, injuries, and deformities

surgeon, general surgeon who specializes in the surgical treatment of more than one body area or system

surgeon, oral dentist who specializes in the surgical treatment of diseases, injuries, and deformities of the mouth

surgery department department providing diagnosis and treatment through surgical procedures

surgical suite one or more operating rooms plus necessary adjunct facilities, such as scrub room(s), recovery room(s), sterile storage area See also *operating room*

surgical technician See *operating room technician*

swing bed See *bed, swing*

Tt

TB unit See *tuberculosis unit*
teaching hospital See *hospital, teaching*
team leader See *nursing team leader*
team nurse See *nurse, team*
team nursing method of organizing nursing services within an inpatient care unit by which groups of registered nurses and auxiliary nursing personnel implement total nursing care programs planned by the team leader for designated patients for the duration of one shift
telecommunications department department providing for management and maintenance of telephone, paging, and disaster communications systems See also *engineering and maintenance department*
telecommunications manager person who plans and directs a hospital's telephone and paging services and telephone and equipment maintenance
tertiary care provision by a large medical center, usually serving a region or state and having sophisticated technological and support facilities, of highly specialized medical and surgical care for unusual and complex medical problems
therapeutic recreation specialist person who assists patients in their recovery or rehabilitation after physical or emotional illness or disability and/or who plans and supervises recreation programs for total patient populations
thermal unit See *burn care unit*
third-party payer party to an insurance or prepayment agreement—usually an insurance company, prepayment plan, or government agency—responsible for paying to the provider designated expenses incurred on behalf of the insured
tissue committee committee composed of medical staff members whose purpose is to evaluate the appropriateness of surgical procedures in the hospital by examination of tissues removed by surgery

training coordinator See *education, director of*
transfer agreement written hospital agreement between two health care institutions for transfer of patients from one to another and for the orderly exchange of pertinent clinical information on patients transferred
transfer, discharge discharge of a patient from one health care institution with arrangements made for the patient's transfer to another health care institution
transfer, intrahospital formal transfer of an inpatient, usually during a single hospitalization, from one nursing care unit, clinical service, or attending physician to another
trauma center service providing emergency and specialized intensive care to critically ill and injured patients See also *emergency service, hospital*
trauma registry data on the incidence, diagnosis, and treatment of acute trauma victims treated in the emergency department
trauma unit See *trauma center*
triage sorting or classification of patients according to the nature or degree of their injury or illness
trustee member of a hospital governing body See also *governing body*
tuberculosis unit unit for treatment of patients with tuberculosis See also *respiratory diseases unit*
tumor registry repository of data drawn from medical records on the incidence of cancer and personal characteristics, treatment, and treatment outcomes of cancer patients

Uu

ultrasound, diagnostic imaging technique used to visualize internal body structures for diagnostic purposes by means of recording reflected acoustic waves above the range of human hearing

uncompensated care those services provided by a hospital or by a physician or other health care professional for which no charge is made or for which no payment is expected

uniform reporting reporting of financial and service data in conformance with prescribed standard definitions to permit comparisons among hospitals

unit area of a hospital that is staffed and equipped for treatment of patients with a specific condition or with other common characteristics

unit clerk person who performs routine clerical and reception tasks in an inpatient care unit

unit manager person who supervises and coordinates administrative management functions for one or more inpatient care units

unrestricted funds See *funds, unrestricted*

UR See *review, utilization*

urologist physician who specializes in the diagnosis and treatment of diseases, injuries, and abnormalities of the urinary tract and urogenital tract

utilization review See *review, utilization*

utilization review committee committee composed of medical staff members whose purpose is to evaluate the appropriateness of admissions, the medical and support services rendered, and the length of stay of patients

utilization review coordinator person who coordinates the utilization review activities of a hospital's medical record department and other departments and who acts as liaison with community agencies concerned with utilization review See also *review, utilization*

vocational rehabilitation counselor See *rehabilitation counselor*

voluntary hospital See *hospital, voluntary*

voluntary hospital system nationwide complex of autonomous, self-established, and self-supported private not-for-profit and investor-owned hospitals in the United States

volunteer person who serves a hospital without pay, such as an in-service volunteer, auxiliary member, or governing board member

volunteer, in-service person who serves a hospital without financial remuneration and who, under the direction of the volunteer services department, or, in cases where there is no volunteer services committee, augments but does not replace paid personnel and professional staff

volunteer services department department of the hospital responsible for coordination of the volunteer services provided in the institution and in institution-based programs

volunteers, director of person who is accountable to administration and who plans, administers, and coordinates a hospital's volunteer services department

ward clerk See *unit clerk*

ward manager See *unit manager*

ward hospital room designed and equipped to house more than four inpatients

wholistic health See *holistic health*

x-ray technologist See *radiologic technologist*

x-ray therapy treatment of disease by means of roentgen rays